I0410180

DO YOU HAVE THE COURAGE TO CHANGE?

The 12 Basic Reasons Why People Don't Change And How You Can

By

DR. WALTER J. URBAN

This book is a work of non-fiction. Names and places have been changed to protect the privacy of all individuals. The events and situations are true.

© 2004 by Dr. Walter J. Urban. All rights reserved.

No part of this book may be reproduced, stored in a retrieval system, or transmitted by any means, electronic, mechanical, photocopying, recording, or otherwise, without written permission from the author.

ISBN: 1-4140-2302-2 (e-book)
ISBN: 1-4140-2301-4 (Paperback)
ISBN: 1-4140-2300-6 (Dust Jacket)

Library of Congress Control Number: 2003098772

This book is printed on acid free paper.

Printed in the United States of America
Bloomington, IN

1stBooks - rev. 04/28/04

FOREWORD

As I see clients on a daily basis and teach throughout the world, I find that many health disorders were caused by daily living patterns and a lack of responsibility for one's way of life. I have been a health and lifestyle "coach" for twenty years and have endeavored to teach people how to be happy and well. The sad thing I have found is that most people truly don't know how. We go innocently through our lives eating harmful foods, not getting enough rest, creating unnecessary stress, and usually don't have a clue that these things can create illness. Until one day, we wake up with an ache here and a pain there and wonder where it came from! Wouldn't it be nice to know ahead of time how to live a long life, free from sickness, preventing trouble before it arrives? Now, finally, Dr. Walter J. Urban has written a simple, step-by-step handbook teaching us about the habits that can create problems in our worlds. He shows us "the twelve basic reasons why people don't change."

Change seems to be the single hardest thing for humans to accomplish in their lives. I was walking through a hospital ward and stopped to talk with a lady with lung cancer who was smoking. I asked her why she would still smoke if she knew it was ruining her lungs and would finally take her life. She told me she would never stop smoking because the habit was stronger than her will to live. Having *the will to live* is crucial! We must create a life that brings us such joy that we can't wait for each day to approach. We must realize that this is truly possible. Could it be that within us lies the power to do this?

This straightforward book gives the keys to unlocking the reasons why we don't change and provides clear steps that show how we can. The reader will benefit from the same professional expertise that thousands of Dr. Urban's clients experienced during his many years of clinical practice. He is a remarkable man who lives and practices the principles he writes about. At 71 years young, he exudes radiant health, with clear skin, strong body, and sparkling eyes. He works long hours either writing or working outside on his ranch or in his organic garden. People half his age have trouble keeping up with him!

We need to wake up and realize how important it is to participate in our own level of wellness. Doctors' offices and hospitals are filled with victims who want a quick fix. Many of the antibiotics are no longer working because we have abused the use of them for so long. Strains of viruses are appearing that are resistant to all antibiotics. Eating healthfully and living a life of less stress can create strong bodies with powerful immunity. The World Health Organization has now defined health as the active state of physical, emotional, mental, and social well being—much more than just the absence of illness.

This book is a practical expression of ways we can empower ourselves to take our lives and our health into our own hands. In it the reader will learn to uncover the hidden reasons behind daily rituals that can lead to a painful existence and learn ways to bring positive change.

Ellen Tart-Jensen, Ph.D., D.Sc.

DEDICATION

This book is dedicated to you, yes you, who want to improve your health by facing all the obstacles you give yourself to achieve your goal.

ACKNOWLEDGMENTS

Ina R. Threatt, Ph.D., told me to sit down and write *this* book. I followed her advice; to Muriel L. Reiffe who typed the manuscript; to Larry "Stroke" Farrel for the excellent illustrations; to all my patients who contributed to my understanding; and to the National Psychological Association for Psychoanalysis where I trained.

PREFACE

For many years I have helped people change, and have realized how difficult it was for them to change. Changing beliefs and habit patterns presents a great challenge even if you are going to die with cardiovascular disease or cancer. Most people are unable to face themselves honestly, much less face actual change. Personal rigidity compounded by commercial propaganda creates a great obstacle. As a psychoanalyst and psychotherapist, and as a consultant to businesses, I have come across various reasons why people don't change. I hope that looking at some of these reasons will serve to help people identify in themselves those particular things that will enable them to get a better perspective so that they may live a healthier and longer life.

As we know, understanding alone is not enough to create change. Positive action must take place. One of my former patients, after several years of psychoanalytic psychotherapy, understood and could recite his entire history, including the psychodynamic relationships, causes and symptoms, as well as other pertinent information. He had reached a point of being able to understand his dreams with very little help from me; however, he kept repeating behavior patterns again and again. He became more and more frustrated because he began to feel he wasn't getting anywhere different in his life. When I asked him when he was going to do things differently, he explained that he thought that things would change by themselves now that he understood things. When this resistance to positive action was uncovered, he got the idea and finally changed his behavior quite rapidly and became so intensely motivated that he accomplished things beyond his dreams.

With this example in mind, I return to the point of the need for positive actions to create change. Some types of change appear to take place automatically in human physiology and in nature. However, we know there is always some type of action involved on an atomic or subatomic level. Thus, the following book is written to promote action on the reader's part.

Action requires the use of the mind and emotions, or a combination of both. As we know, the mind has many levels according to psychoanalytic theory: the conscious, the preconscious and the unconscious. The word subconscious is frequently used in everyday language to refer to the unconscious. Therefore understanding how the mind works is basic to achieving changes or preventing change. A similar situation exists for emotions that may effect change. As the mind and emotions interact the situation may become more complicated; for example, fear may prevent rational and logical thinking and behavior.

The need to free oneself from behavior that is determined by unconscious needs is of great importance, so that rational choices can be made in the service of good health. To free oneself, the unconscious must be made conscious, so that full awareness occurs which can be followed by positive rational action that breaks old habit patterns that are self-destructive.

With the aforementioned in mind, let's look at why change is necessary to live a long, healthy life. The main treatment tools of western medicine are drugs and surgery to treat symptoms of disease processes. Not enough attention is paid to the underlying causes of disease. The world we live in becomes more polluted each year. The air, water and soil are basic to life, but have indirectly become a source contributing to premature death.

Other sources of pollution that get little recognition are positive ions coming from electricity and subatomic radiation from video display terminals (VDTs) such as televisions and computers.

Many books have been written about "how to" do different things. However, understanding why people don't change is rarely written about. People don't change because of many reasons. It is these very reasons that prevent change from taking place. Once these reasons are looked at clearly and understood as obstacles to change, changing becomes easier to accomplish. Very often there is a combination of obstacles, which tend to reinforce each other, thus making change a very difficult task. If these obstacles or reasons are understood one by one, the roadblocks to change can be broken down into their component parts and successfully overcome.

It is easy to tell someone "how to" do something. However, proper understanding of what is preventing them from doing what they rationally want to do, is very important. With this in mind, the chapters in this book look at some of the major reasons that act as obstacles to change.

When you read this book, use it as a tool to examine yourself and see if any of the concepts apply to you. If there is something you are trying to change, whether it be to improve your diet, to exercise regularly, or to improve your finances, see which chapter or combination of chapters applies to the specific issue that you want to change. Remember, if you understand what is in your way to getting to your goal, it is easier to get there. Using this book will require you to think more about yourself, rather than provide a quick "how to" formula. Stick to your job of self-examination and you will achieve your goals.

TABLE OF CONTENTS

THE TEN BELIEFS THAT MAY SHORTEN YOUR LIFE

1. The Food and Drug Administration (FDA) is protecting your health and the Environmental Protection Agency (EPA) is doing all it can to protect your health.

2. Genetically engineered (G.E.) food will help you and your children.

3. Pharmaceutical companies and their products are in business to help you.

4. Always treat the symptom with drugs; pay no attention to the cause of disease.

5. The American Cancer Society and the National Cancer Institute will find the cause of cancer and are not financially and politically controlled.

6. Radiation and chemotherapy are good therapies for cancer.

7. Milk and milk products are good for you and your children.

8. The more money you have, the healthier you will become.

9. It's okay to eat food with herbicides, insecticides and fungicides; fertilizers and toxic chemicals; animal drugs (antibiotics, hormones, veterinary medicines—200 active ingredients); food additives (300 colorings, preservatives, waxes, flavorings, emulsifiers, etc.) and processing aids and contaminants (10,000 solvents, resins, etc.)

10. Your body will be unaffected by everything you put into it (conventionally grown and processed food and genetically engineered food and fish), as long as you don't think about it.

IT'S UP TO YOU

What you can do

Is up to you

Want to live long

Sing nature's song

Then you will achieve

No more need to grieve

The more you will do

The better for you

If you start today

You will make your way

Your children you will save

No longer be a slave

To false information

Misleading the nation

Wake up your mind

Truth you will find

Become more aware

You are getting there

Learning prevention
Freeing your tension
Lifting your spirit
Listen and hear it
Do all you can
Make a good plan
What you can do
Is up to you.

START IMPROVING
YOUR HEALTH NOW

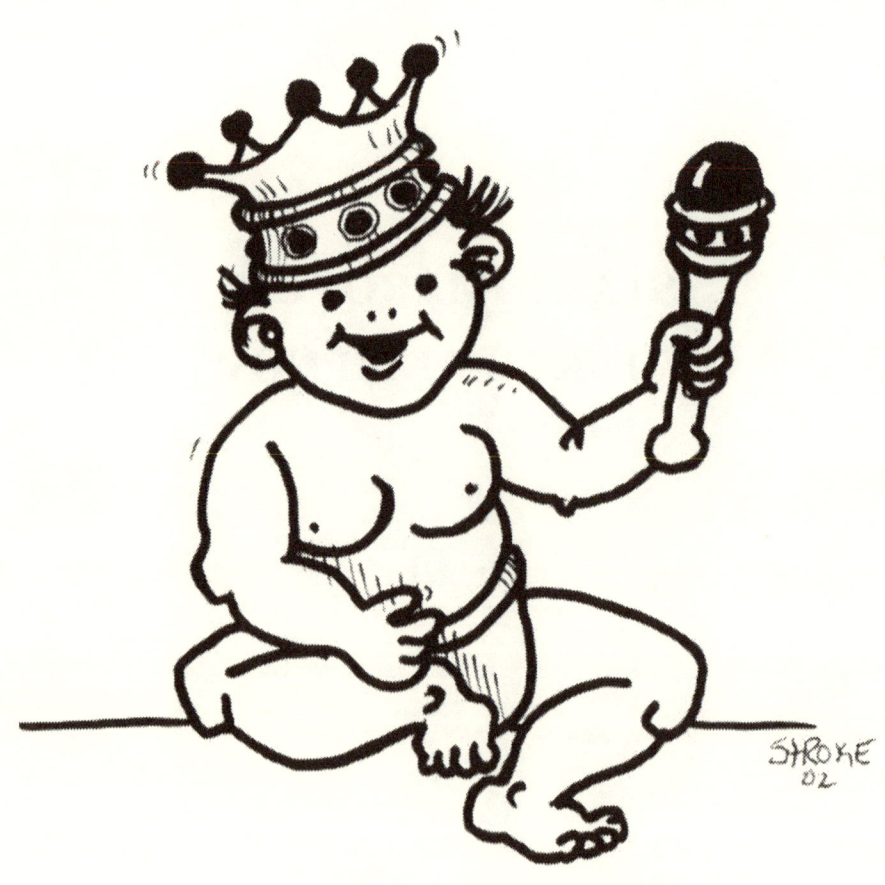

UNCONSCIOUS OMNIPOTENCE

CHAPTER ONE

UNCONSCIOUS OMNIPOTENCE

When you hear about other people dying of heart attacks, strokes or cancer, do you think it can happen to you or do you think you won't be a victim? Most people think it will never happen to them; terminal diseases only happen to others. You think you feel good, you're "eating healthy" and getting some exercise. Do you know the statistics? Cardiovascular disease is the number one deadly disease in the United States, and according to the American Cancer Society the life risk for cancer for American males is 1 out of 2, and for females, 1 out of 3. Childhood cancer is rising. Somehow, you still believe it will be someone else who dies prematurely and not you.

You are convinced you are invulnerable or don't even bother to think about terminal illness. Your mind is occupied with daily life and you give little thought to the strong possibility that you will die prematurely.

Why is this a common belief in many people? I remember the grief of one of my former patients whose 42-year-old brother who was a weight lifter and athlete suddenly died of a heart attack. My patient was in shock for several days and couldn't believe her strong brother had died. My patient told me how her brother used to jog several times a week and how energetic and robust he was. No thought was ever given to the possibility that he could even get sick, much less die suddenly of a heart attack.

Many people simply assume that nothing will ever happen to them. They never even think about such a tragic possibility and continue living the lifestyle that they live. Many of these people think they are strong and powerful without any realization of their true state of health. Many of these people don't even bother to have a thorough blood analysis to get a clinical picture of what is really going on.

Why is this so? This is where the concept of unconscious omnipotence may very well play a role. Many people believe they are all powerful or omnipotent; however, they do not have a clear and conscious awareness of this belief. How does this kind of belief develop? It goes back to infancy and childhood. When we are born all our needs are usually taken care of. We are fed, cleaned and provided for. The infant doesn't have to do anything to receive this basic nurturing; it simply has to exist. If something is wrong, the infant may cry and will usually receive immediate attention. Since it can only lie on its back in the early stages, its helplessness requires the caretaker to do everything for it. The infant perceives its world as if it is powerful enough to have all its needs taken care of, and continues to experience itself as the center of the world. The caretaker comes to it and brings it food, cleans it, etc. This concept of being powerful grows during infancy and very early childhood, when it may be reinforced by parental actions. The concept of omnipotence grows in the psyche of the child. Little by little it gains in strength and forms a belief in the mind of the growing child.

As the child continues to grow older and meets frustrating circumstances as well as reality limitations, it learns that it cannot have its way in getting all its needs and desires satisfied as it did in infancy. The growing child and adolescent continues to be confronted with reality, and begins to realize more and more that it is not all powerful in the face of the external world. The adolescent and adult begin to adjust more and more to how the world really is, and learns to cope with its frustrations, impasses and limits. Eventually the original omnipotence that it experienced as an infant and very young child becomes forgotten and is buried deep in the psyche and becomes unconscious. The omnipotence is unconscious, but not dead. That is, it still lives in the mind and can influence the present adult state of affairs. Its influence makes the adult think in certain ways, which in turn creates certain behavior(s) in the adult. For example, it may lead to unrealistic beliefs, such as, "I will never get a heart attack" or "I know what you are thinking."

This buried or unconscious omnipotent belief can cause a great number of problems in one's life and can be considered a normal phenomenon, since most people have this core belief about themselves. Until this is made conscious either by self-analysis (if possible) or psychotherapy, the belief will continue to have an influence on one's life. The danger is that it can create unrealistic ideas or behavior, as in a thrill seeker who believes that diving off the mountain into the water is perfectly safe.

An interesting example of unconscious omnipotence working in combination with aggression is a former client of mine. Let's call him Joe. At age 19 he was expelled from college for drinking and fighting. During the first visit to my office at a mental health center he pushed the desk in front of me, trying to pin me to the wall. He had a part-time job driving a truck and had had six accidents in a three-month period. He always had to be first. During one visit, he asked me if I had heard the news about him on the radio. He had gone skydiving and had landed on someone's roof. During another visit he proudly told me how he had told the state police to pull over because they were driving with their bright lights on and didn't turn them off when he signaled them. These examples of his behavior were all manifestations of how powerful he felt as well as how angry he was. During the time of the Kennedy assassination he told me about the telescope he had and his high-powered rifle. I will always remember walking out of my office building in New York and visually checking the rooftops for several weeks. The purpose here is to illustrate, rather than to discuss the therapy of my former client. However, as a matter of interest, when he terminated therapy he was a successful owner of his own company as well as of a thirty foot yacht! He was extremely polite, respectful and had a satisfying relationship with his girlfriend. He no longer wanted to kill his father, and we looked back and laughed at his former behavior.

Another example of omnipotence at work and this time not completely unconscious, was a student of mine. Bill believed that cars were in his way and that the drivers were just stupid. This wasn't just one or two other cars, but many cars that interfered with his driving every day. He would curse them instantly and believed the roadway had to be cleared for him. On one occasion a big truck was turning into the road he needed and was ahead of him. There was no way to pass the truck on this one-lane road so he decided to get to my office another way. He got lost and came one and one-half hours late because he took the wrong road. I asked him, upon arrival, why he didn't use the map and he said he didn't need a map. He thought he could find his own way. I told him he would have been much better off with the map. Bill responded by saying those roads weren't on the map. I told him that they *were* on the map, and then he realized how he had defended his position in an irrational way.

Further, Bill believed he knew what the stock market was going to do tomorrow and that he plans to make millions of dollars in 6 months starting with $3,000. An obvious case of omnipotence for a man who was educated as an engineer. Bill also believed that smoking cigarettes would not hurt his lungs because he lifted weights and jogged and was very strong. How can an educated man deny reality so much? The answer: OMNIPOTENCE!

What You Can Do

Realize that you are not omnipotent and that you can be vulnerable to cardiovascular disease, cancer or any other illness. Be sure to be aware of the reality consequences of your behavior and that the law of cause and effect will take place. No person is all-powerful. Be aware of the "omnipotent child" in you who may influence your thinking and behavior.

Exercise

Examine your beliefs. Do you think you will never have a serious illness? Do you need to be first when driving? Do you ever think you are invulnerable or extremely powerful? Do you think you are superior to people around you? Do you want to be given special treatment? If you answered YES to any question, reread the chapter and repeat the exercise in one week.

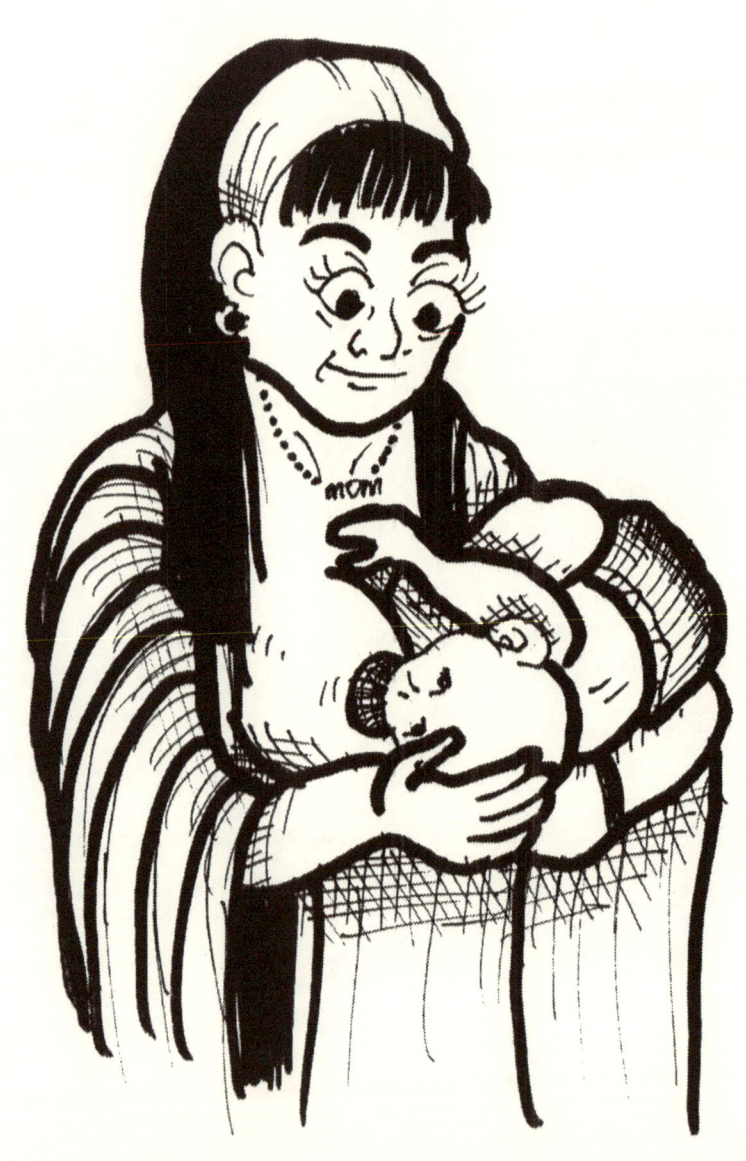

MOMMY, MOMMY

CHAPTER TWO

MOMMY, MOMMY

Did you ever wish to come home from work and have dinner waiting for you? Some of us are fortunate enough for dinner to be there. Most of us have to make our own dinner or eat out. It is much easier to eat out than prepare our own meal. The evidence is there for eating out. Billions of hamburgers have been sold. Millions of chicken parts have been sold; millions of tacos have been sold by the fast food chains. Let's not leave out the pizzas.

Just think of the hormones, antibiotics, pesticides, fried oils, salt, white flour and other chemicals that are eaten. After all, it's quicker and easier to fill your stomach with burgers, fries, fried chicken, pizzas, and tacos rather than to fill it with healthy organic food. Let's not forget the soft drinks that usually go with the fast food that contain sugar, sweeteners, caffeine, as well as the bubbly gas which is made with carbon dioxide that is a human waste product that we exhale.

So here you have it. Fast food and a drink probably cost more than a salad that you make at home. So the question is, why do we knowingly eat things that diminish our health? Why is it so hard to prepare more of our food at home?

We usually tell ourselves different reasons such as we worked hard all day, we are tired, we didn't have the time to shop, it's inconvenient, etc. All these reasons may be true; however, there may be an underlying reason that we are not so conscious of. Sure we would like dinner as well as other meals prepared for us. Even Mom would like to be served, yet she has to serve the children, so she may take them out for fast food and drink.

If you measure the time it takes to get to the fast food, the time you wait, the time you eat and get home, you may find it actually takes less time to prepare food at home. However, home preparation takes work that you may not want to do, whereas the restaurant trip seems to be easier. What is behind all of this self-destructive eating of fast foods?

After all, we know what we are doing. We know that a fast food meal is unhealthy. Somehow we cannot stop ourselves despite our rational evaluation.

Some of us never get over the wish to be taken care of. However, this wish may not be conscious. If we prepare the meal at home, we have to do the work and be the caregiver; if we eat out the food preparation is done for us. The wish to be taken care of goes back to infancy and childhood when we hopefully were taken care of. However this wish is never outgrown in many of us. We are still seeking a mothering figure, hence the chapter title, "Mommy, Mommy."

Yes, some of us are still seeking Mommy, but we are usually unaware of this as adults. We give ourselves many reasons to justify fast food, but rarely get at the deeper understanding of some of our true motives. After all, as we become more informed about health, why is the fast food industry continuing to grow? Why can't we put our knowledge of good health into use? Perhaps we are being controlled by our unconscious wish to be taken care of by Mommy, rather than being the rational adult. Does this make any sense to you? Why not experiment with yourself and find out how you feel and think just before you are ready for the fast food meal, and then try to prepare your meal at home and see what you experience. Put your timer on and see how long it takes to prepare at home and compare it to the fast food trip time.

Janet, a beautiful 29 year old woman with two children ages 5 and 7, was unhappily married. I met her while waiting to have the oil changed in my car. We chatted and became friends. She was very much interested in health and nutrition and was quite knowledgeable about healthy eating. She was in the process of moving to a new house and quite busy packing. She told me she took her children to eat hamburgers even though she knew better. She said she had to be a mother to her husband, whom she resented. She wanted to leave the marriage but stayed for the children. She went out to eat frequently and ate "bad food" because she did not have the patience to prepare food at home. She wanted someone to serve her, not to be the one who had to do the preparation and serving. She wished her husband would do something when he came home from work other than watch TV. She had the children all day and wanted relief. Instead she had to keep being the caretaker, so to make it easier for herself she would take the children out and let her husband fend for himself for dinner. She ate her fast food telling herself she knew she shouldn't be eating it. Janet wanted to be mothered herself and have a long break from being the mother to her children and husband. She was seeking Mommy, because aside from the reality of her mothering responsibilities to her children, she was not fully grown up herself. Does this sound familiar? Are you looking for Mommy too?

What you can do

Be aware of your wish to be taken care of but don't let it make decisions for you by eating fast food. Staying healthy takes your effort and "mommy" is no longer there for you. As an adult you must take care of yourself and use the knowledge you have to maintain good health.

Exercise

Try not eating out for two weeks. Prepare all your meals including lunch. Do more things for yourself and give yourself three chores a week that will make you more self-reliant. Buy a juicer and make yourself fresh vegetable juice Saturday and Sunday. If you haven't done these things in the next two weeks, try again or go home to Mommy.

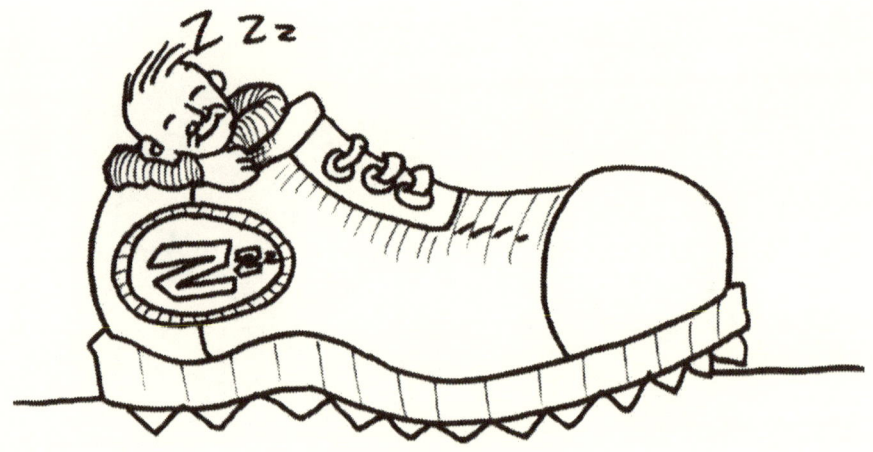

THE OLD SHOE

CHAPTER THREE

THE OLD SHOE

You've probably heard some saying about "the old shoe is comfortable." When you get new shoes, it takes a bit of time till you break them in and they become as comfortable as the old ones. This is nothing new to you; however, the comfort you may be seeking may have detrimental aspects. Did you ever continue to stay with something because it was the easiest and most comfortable way? We tend to be "creatures of habit" and often repeat things again and again and form habit patterns.

These comfortable habits may have to do with anything in your life such as food, clothes, sleeping, job, finances, personal relationships, etc. Sometimes habits can be rewarding if they are positive ones, such as brushing your teeth after every meal. However, having orange juice (bottled or frozen), eggs, bacon, toast with butter or jelly and coffee for breakfast every morning may not be the best habit to keep repeating. So it is the nature of the habit that needs to be looked at.

You need to examine all your activities and evaluate whether they are constructive or self-destructive. The ones that you know are self destructive are obviously the ones you may consider for elimination. However, these activities or habits may have a very comforting factor for you. Your comfort and repetition may be something you **don't** want to give up. Why give up something you know for something you don't know? You probably don't know what it's like to be without this particular habit and don't know what a healthier habit is like. If you drink a cup of coffee every morning to help to start the day and try going without it or substitute non-caffeinated tea, you're taking a risk and leaving the comfort zone. A risk you may not be prepared to take! On the other hand, maybe a risk, which would help you improve.

When we look behind the comfort zone we usually find two things, insecurity and fear. We usually find that insecurity and fear have a relationship with each other. Very often insecurity develops out of fear. Let's look at a simple example of an unhappy mate who doesn't leave the relationship because of insecurity. The pros and cons have been evaluated and the "bad" times are much greater than the "good" times in the relationship. Logic says after years of trying to "work it out" or "fix" it, it isn't getting any better. He or she can't leave because it may be worse out of the relationship. Being "alone" makes the person feel insecure. Perhaps, on another deeper level, the person is "afraid" to be alone i.e. without this particular mate. So the choice of leaving is not made, and the fear of being alone is the deciding factor. This may or may not be in the consciousness of the person. In any case, the effect may be the same. Do nothing; just keep things the way they are. Make no decision; stay "comfortable." Of course the person isn't really comfortable in this case, since there is a conflict. However, the person is more comfortable in the old shoe than thinking about making a decision. Finding a new relationship at age X and not getting any younger or trimmer may be quite risky. By the way, if there are any children involved, this may be another reason to consider. What will happen to them? What about their lives?

Let's look at the underlying issues of insecurity and fear. Both have many aspects that may deal with the past, present or future and any combination thereof. For example insecurity may go back to infancy, childhood, adolescence, or past adult life. Lack of developing adequate or good security may stem from a variety of reasons or combination of things, dating back to inadequate nurturing as an infant or in childhood. Difficult and/or traumatic experiences in adolescence and in adult life may also lead to insecurity, especially if the earlier years did not have a good secure foundation. Both the present situation and/or environment, which has current threats, may help create insecurity. Future uncertainties such as the loss of a job or a potential loss of a significant person, as well as many other circumstances, may help create insecurity. A person's own personality may also be a precursor to insecurity. For example, lack of sufficient self-esteem or confidence can increase vulnerability. As you can see there are innumerable things that feed insecurity, thus contributing to the desire to keep things as they are; that is, comfortable.

Now let's have a brief look at fear. Fear may stem from many things. It may come from a threat, which the person believes may be or is too great to cope with. The person may feel or may have felt in the past that he or she was overwhelmed or could be overwhelmed. Underlying fear, like insecurity, may stem from any time or aspect of the person's life, as well as anticipated or upcoming events. Possibilities of fear-producing events, circumstances and environments are too numerous to mention, and vary from person to person.

With insecurity and fear as underlying issues in a person's makeup, staying comfortable in the old shoe often serves as an important obstacle to change. When you know what you've got and don't know what you're going to get, or if you are going to get anything at all, when you let go of the old shoe, it's often easier to do nothing. Think about it and see if this old shoe fits you.

What you can do

If you stay comfortable in your "old shoe" you'll never get a new pair. Think of yourself as having the courage to leave your comfort zone and start with a small new step. Step by step you can walk yourself anywhere and your courage will build and your insecurity will diminish. Visualize yourself in your "new shoes" and saying goodbye to the old ones.

Exercise

Do one new thing every day for two weeks. Change some part of your daily routine. Eat only fruits and vegetables for one day a week for two weeks. Stop drinking coffee for three consecutive days twice in two weeks. Meditate for ten minutes every day for two weeks. If you have succeeded, congratulate yourself; if you haven't, ask yourself why you fear change.

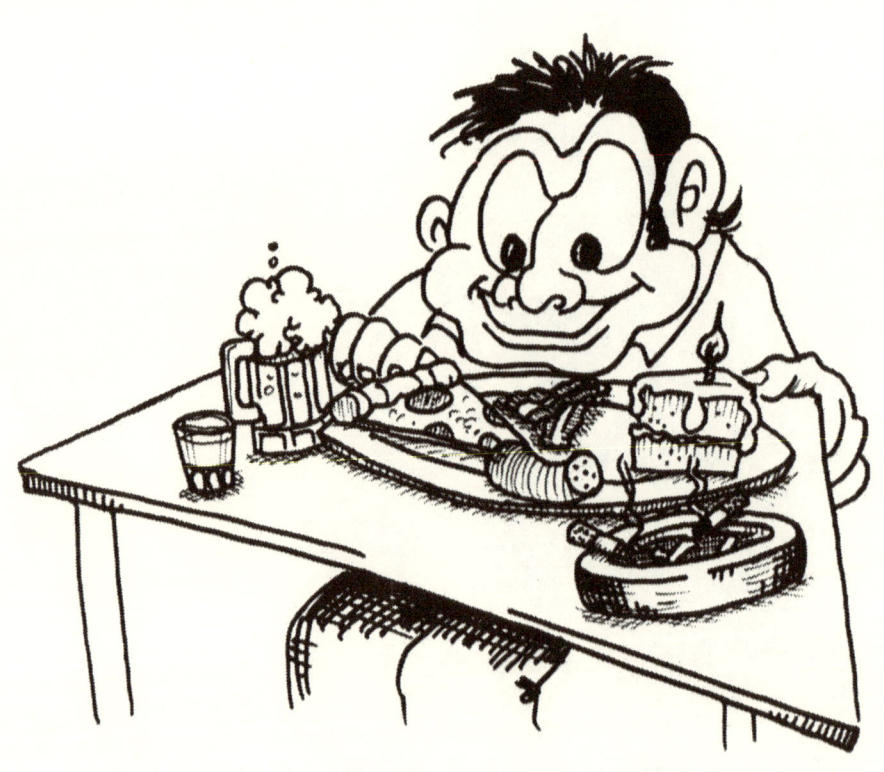

A LITTLE BIT

CHAPTER FOUR

A LITTLE BIT

Did you ever say to yourself, "It's okay" because you only had a little bit of pizza, coke and French fries? Just a little bit of ice cream, cake, chocolate, candy, wine, beer, fried food, hard liquor, white flour, hamburgers, food coloring, whipped cream, food additive, pesticide, fertilizer, tap water, caffeine, nicotine, drugs (legal or illegal), etc., can add up over the years and have a cumulative effect. How about just a little bit of unprotected sex? How about just a little bit over the speed limit, or a very little bit of thrill-seeking with sky diving, bungee jumping, etc.?

What is behind the idea of having just a little bit of something that you know may not be the best choice for you? Let's look at three things that may be part of the issue that allows you to justify to yourself that a little bit is okay. The first issue may be having pleasure. You really enjoy your morning cup of coffee. You only put in a little bit of cream (or cream substitute) and sugar. For some of you, it's the taste and/or the smell. For others, it's because it gets you going because you didn't have enough sleep, or you'd rather not face the day so you don't really want to get up. Sometimes you need a little bit more coffee during the day to keep you going, or perhaps a little bit of coke to get you going. I remember, when I consulted in New York City, riding up the elevator in the morning with several people carrying their large coffee cups with them. They were sipping the coffee. They couldn't wait to get to the coffee machine at work. The boss had his own expresso machine in his private kitchen.

Remember, the first source of pleasure in life was probably being nurtured at the breast for most of you. Food usually remains as a primary source of pleasure. So why not give yourself a little bit of pleasure in your life? After all, life can be a struggle for many of us. Life has its stress, chores and requires work. So a little bit of pleasurable indulgence is needed by many to keep going.

As you repeat these personal pleasures they form habits, and some may actually became addictions. Addictions are the second reason behind these little or maybe not-so-little pleasures. Addictions may be physical, psychological/ emotional or any combination thereof. We know that nicotine is physically addictive. You may also be a sugar addict. How about the possibility of a personal relationship in which logic tells you it's not right, but your emotional and/or physical pleasure keeps you addicted? A friend of mine usually has a major fight with his girlfriend every weekend when he sees her. He always tells me that the relationship is over. "It's the end." However, he's back with her the next weekend. This pattern has been going on for almost the two years that I know him. Does this sound familiar?

Very often addictions have deep roots and may stem from early life experiences that helped develop addictions. These early experiences vary from person to person. Think about your past and investigate for yourself. Did you ever have a cup of hot chocolate as a child and did it make you feel good? Of course as a child you didn't know that a quick sugar fix was the foundation for your present pleasure. Your adult knowledge tells you that sugar is not good for you, so you only have a little bit!

The third issue is pain; that is, the avoidance of pain. None of us (who are healthy) are interested in feeling pain. We try to avoid pain in any way we can. Some people eat, drink, smoke, take drugs, etc., to avoid pain, and perhaps have a little pleasure at the same time. That morning cup of coffee may alleviate the pain of feeling tired and having to get up to face the day. The smell, the taste and the caffeine boost all come from that one cup of coffee. Some of us feel anxiety, stress, depression, sadness, loneliness or other uncomfortable emotional states. When we feel these different types of pain we want relief, and we do things that help us remove and get away from the pain. Perhaps a little bit of alcohol or sugar. Many of us turn to the original nurturing satisfier, food.

Now when we put these three: pleasure, addictions, and the avoidance of pain, together, they have a powerful effect on us. Some of us have all three reasons and they tend to reinforce each other. It's not surprising that we allow ourselves to have a little bit of whatever makes us feel better. We believe a little bit won't hurt and does the immediate job. After years of "a little bit," it is no longer a little bit.

What about considering learning to have pleasure in a healthy way and solving the underlying motivating issues? Working on these things "a little bit" may be more helpful than you realize!

What you can do

Stop and think before you indulge yourself in "a little bit" of what you know is not good for you. Ask yourself what you are trying to achieve by this "little bit" or what you are running away from. When you stay in this moment or these minutes of time, you will make a discovery that will help strengthen you because you will find out something important about yourself.

Exercise

Every time you have a "little bit" of what you know is unhealthy (pizza, coke, fries, cigarettes, candy, cake, ice cream, pie, coffee, bacon, meat, salt, etc.) put $5 in a cup.

Do this for two weeks. If you have over $25 in the cup give it to your mate; if less, keep it.

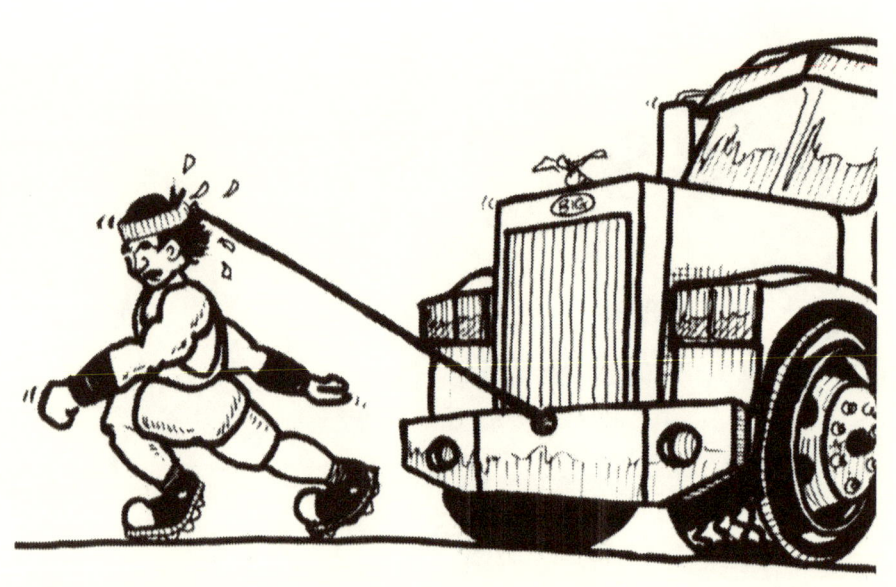

TOO HARD

CHAPTER FIVE

TOO HARD

Did you ever get the feeling or the idea that something was too hard to do? Well you are not alone. Many of us have had the same thought: it's too hard. When we think that something is too hard to do, we make that thought come true because either we never try to do it or predetermine that we can't do it. Thinking it's too hard makes it too hard for us to proceed. Perhaps you set an unrealistic goal such as exercising 6 hours a week, or giving up coffee tomorrow, or painting a picture, or stopping smoking, or learning to play chess, or studying one stock for an hour, or whatever.

You create a mindset when you say, "it's too hard." That mindset which you create becomes your boss. In essence you are giving up. You forget to break down the task into very small components that you can succeed with. You probably could learn one new word of Chinese every day if it were important to you and you were motivated. Chances are that your first response to learning Chinese would be that it's too hard to do. Who makes things too hard to do? You do. Of course you always have a good reason to justify your position. So you go on living your lifestyle without undertaking those tasks that you know would be good for you and most likely better your life.

Helene had a Keogh plan and two mutual funds. She didn't even know the details of what was in the plan and couldn't remember the names of the mutual funds. She didn't know exactly how much she started with and had no idea of their present value because she hadn't checked them for the last year and a half. It was too much trouble to do and it would be too hard to research what would work best, given the current market conditions, which keep changing. She complained of always just getting by financially even though she had a very good salary and her Keogh and mutual funds were very important to her. It was too hard to keep track of her money and too hard to know exactly where all her salary went. Sound familiar?

Now take Sandy who owned two stocks. She forgot the purchase price of each stock and rarely knew the daily trading price. Was it too hard to keep track of two stocks? I guess it was for Sandy.

Now take Boris, a Russian immigrant who speaks fluent English, learned to scuba dive, sail, lift weights, became a professional photographer and a maker of documentary films, buys and sells cars, became a US citizen and lives close to the beach in Santa Monica, California, one of the most desirable places in the United States. I guess it wasn't too hard for Boris who came to the US on his own with practically no money. Perhaps Boris should meet with Helene and Sandy! Perhaps all three should meet with Kim, who grew up in the ghetto in Indiana, and has a Black Belt and a Ph.D.

People who think it's too hard often say, "I can't." If you listen to someone's use of language, you can usually get a clue to how they think. Listen to your own language and notice if you say, "I can't." If you hear yourself saying it, keep track of how many times a day or week you say it. Saying, "I can't" often means you are predisposed to a sense of failure about whatever you are referring to.

Investigate why you think that way is helpful and be sure not to think "it's too hard" to do!

Sometimes people who say, "I can't," also think, "I can't do it alone." Doing things alone is difficult for many people. Working out at home may be more convenient and less expensive than paying a health club and transportation costs, however, how many people have a home gym? There are many ads in the classified to sell exercise equipment that is almost new. Some people have difficulty or feel uncomfortable about going to a restaurant or movie alone. Others have difficulty living alone. Still others have fear of getting older and being alone.

Many people seek support from others, which is perfectly fine to do. Doing things together often is helpful and the "I can't" may change into "I'll try." People can encourage and help each other as well as learn from each other. What was originally "too hard" becomes easier to face with support. When something is "too hard" perhaps you will be interested in understanding why it is too hard, and why getting support allows you to approach the issue. If you choose to look deeply at yourself, you may discover some of the origins of how you developed the "it's too hard" and "I can't" part of yourself.

What you can do

If you change your thought from "it's too hard" to "I can do it" you are programming yourself for success. When you take the first small achievable step you will overcome your resistance and the ball will start rolling. Set yourself up for success by thinking of yourself as stronger than you used to be.

Exercise

Select three tasks that you've thought were too hard for you to do. Do them in the next week. If you succeed, do three more the second week; if you don't succeed, try them again the third week. Do you feel stronger at the end of the second week or did you give up?

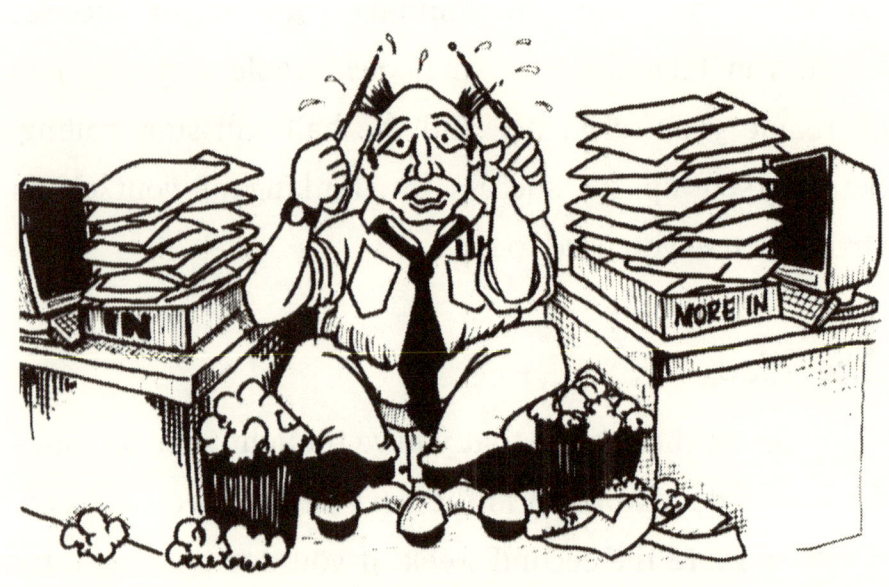

BUSY, BUSY, BUSY

CHAPTER SIX

BUSY, BUSY, BUSY

You get up in the morning, take care of your bathroom activities, get dressed, maybe prepare and eat breakfast, travel to work, and hope to arrive on time if transportation was without problems. This could be considered a typical weekday morning for a majority of you.

Next you get to work and the pressure to produce starts, because in one way or another you are being watched and evaluated whether you are an office worker, engineer, waiter, stockbroker or second vice president. You want to keep your job, or perhaps need to keep your job, so you give it your best, unless you can get away with doing less. Some of you want to advance, so you work every minute to prove yourself. Others couldn't care less.

Next comes lunch break for those of you who don't have a coffee break. Sometimes you have personal things, other than lunch, to do so you eat quickly to make sure to get back on time. Only half a day to go. You slow down about an hour and a half after lunch when the digestion process calls for energy. Of course this varies depending upon what you ate for lunch. Those of you who eat a light meal, such as a large salad, are less tired than the meat eaters.

Soon, but not soon enough, it's time to leave work and rush off, hoping transportation is on time. Those of you who drive are tempted to speed to get home or wherever you're going as fast as possible. In the San Diego area, where I live, the rush hour traffic can be frustrating, not only to speeders, because traffic crawls very slowly. When it finally breaks open you hit the pedal. My car actually appeared to be hardly moving when I drove at 70 mph, the speed limit, when some cars passed me by in a flash. They had been doing 85 to 90.

You get home and you have a list of things to do as well as eat. Everybody's list varies so we don't need to go into details. Those of you with children have some extras to do. You try to get everything done, maybe even exercise or jog, so you can have some time for yourself or "free" time. This rarely happens unless you stay up very late. So you get to bed after preparing for the next day. Your clothes are ready for morning, or they may not be and you may pay the consequences the next morning.

Now let us look at the weekends. If you've been out late and/or drinking Friday night, you'd like a little more sleep Saturday morning. You look forward to the weekend, no job to go to. However, it's time for your "home job" you've got to catch up with innumerable chores, whether it be the laundry, cleaning, the car, the garden, shopping, ironing (if you do any), your personal projects, etc. Saturday night is "your" time; you need some fun and pleasure, not only Friday night. So you let loose and go for it, knowing that you can sleep late on Sunday morning. You may even indulge yourself with pleasure foods on Sunday, knowing Monday is coming. Sunday night you try to get to bed early in preparation for Monday morning.

The above description may not fit all of you, but doesn't it apply to many of you? With this in mind, we can see how busy you are. Yes, you are really busy. Busy, busy, busy! Imagine what it would be like if you had to make changes in this routine. You are so busy, you can't even think about it. Just keeping up with what you have to do is difficult enough. You are so busy all the time, so why think of adding new things to your life?

Very often your busy routine is disturbed because problems come up. For some of us there is a new problem every day. Something always happens. The wife, the husband, the girl- or boyfriend, the car, the kids, a cold, something breaks, the rain or snow, etc.; "it's always something." Problems, problems and more problems. You're alive and problems never stop. Isn't that how life is?

Now between being so busy and taking care of the problems that keep arising, how can you even start doing new things? Is it possible? Many of you are not able to keep up with the way your life is now. If this is how you feel, this may be an obstacle to your changing. Ask yourself if this kind of thinking and living is something you do. If it is, please stop and evaluate it so that you will have more choices in your life. Are you too busy to change?

What you can do

Take a good look at why every minute of your life is filled with things to do. Who makes you so busy that you have no time to think about making beneficial changes? Being busy is not an excuse for living an unhealthy lifestyle. How about getting busy with taking better care of yourself!

Exercise

Every night before you go to bed spend five minutes evaluating the day, five minutes thinking about how you can eliminate what is unnecessary for tomorrow, and five minutes in mental silence. Do this for two weeks and ask yourself if you have become calmer.

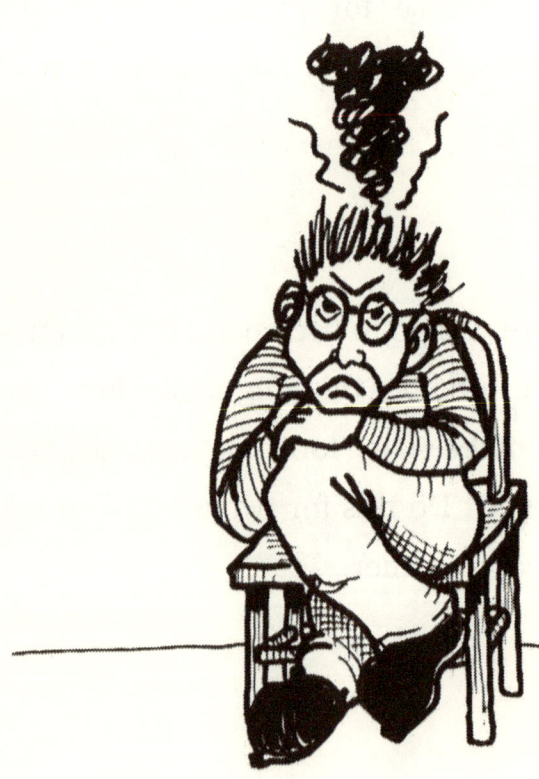

ATTITUDE

CHAPTER SEVEN

ATTITUDE

Little children imitate the behavior of their parents. They learn to speak by repeating what they hear. They learn to eat what their parents eat. Parents become the role models for their children. As the children grow up they often use their role models such as relatives, teachers, peers, idols, etc. This process of using role models takes place by identifying with the other person and is called identification.

As children continue to grow up they also develop attitudes toward different things. These attitudes often influence their thoughts and behavior. After years of repeating certain attitudes toward different things, these attitudes tend to become automatic and part of the personality.

Sometimes people do not realize that they have "an attitude" toward something because their automatic response seems so natural to them. These attitudes play an important role in life and affect the capacity to change. Thoughts such as "Yes, I can" and, "No, I can't" or "Yes, I will" and "No, I won't" may have a major effect upon one's health and well being. "Yes, I can" stop smoking. "No, I can't" stop smoking. "Yes I can exercise every day. "No I can't." "Yes I can drink fresh vegetable juice every day," "No I can't," etc.

Positive and negative attitudes affect almost every area of your life, your personal relationships, your workplace, your diet, your finances, etc. If your attitudes about different things are fixed negatives, your chances of success are greatly reduced. It is important to become aware of what your attitudes are because if you are not, then you are stuck and have little chance of changing. If you automatically have a closed, locked mind, new information cannot come in. You have no way to evaluate what you refuse to think about. Obviously, negative attitudes limit your world of information during this "information age."

I tried telling a relative of mine who needs to lose some weight about the benefits of a detoxification program using colonics. The response I got was, "Don't tell me; I don't want to hear about it." I was a bit shocked since this person is very intelligent and had a career as a teacher. However, the attitude dominated the intellect. Very often, attitude and emotions are so strong that logic and reasoning never have a chance. Many years later I brought up the same subject with this person. Health awareness and detoxification have grown enormously, and I still got the same response. However, this time, with anger and a warning to not ever talk about colonics again.

Look at yourself and see if you have any attitudes that prevent you from improving your life. If you can keep your mind open you will benefit from your positive attitude, rather than shortchange your life by having a negative attitude. There was an old song with the words saying, "accentuate the positive, eliminate the negative, and don't mess with Mr. In-Between." If you have a negative attitude or an "it doesn't matter" outlook, you probably won't have any desire to change. "You can lead a horse to water..." you know the rest.

Some people go beyond having a negative attitude and actually defend what seems like an illogical position. Many years ago I was trying, and I mean *trying* because I did not succeed, to help an acquaintance with information about the contaminants in food. He told me he knew all about it; however, he wasn't going to change his diet because "a little bit of poison is good for you," he said. "It strengthens your system." He was so adamant about his beliefs that I quickly gave up. This was a good learning experience for me because before this I didn't know when to stop trying to convince people to learn about healthy food.

What you can do

Ask yourself if you are aware of your attitude toward specific things. Do you consider your outlook a positive or a negative one? Do you have fixed ideas or are you open to new information? Do you get emotional or defensive when certain topics are discussed? Does your attitude toward food and exercise enhance your health?

Exercise

Ask five people who know you well whether they think your attitude is positive or negative. Pick three experiences that were upsetting and ask yourself what you can learn from them. Look in the mirror and smile, then frown. Repeat this three times and decide which face you like better.

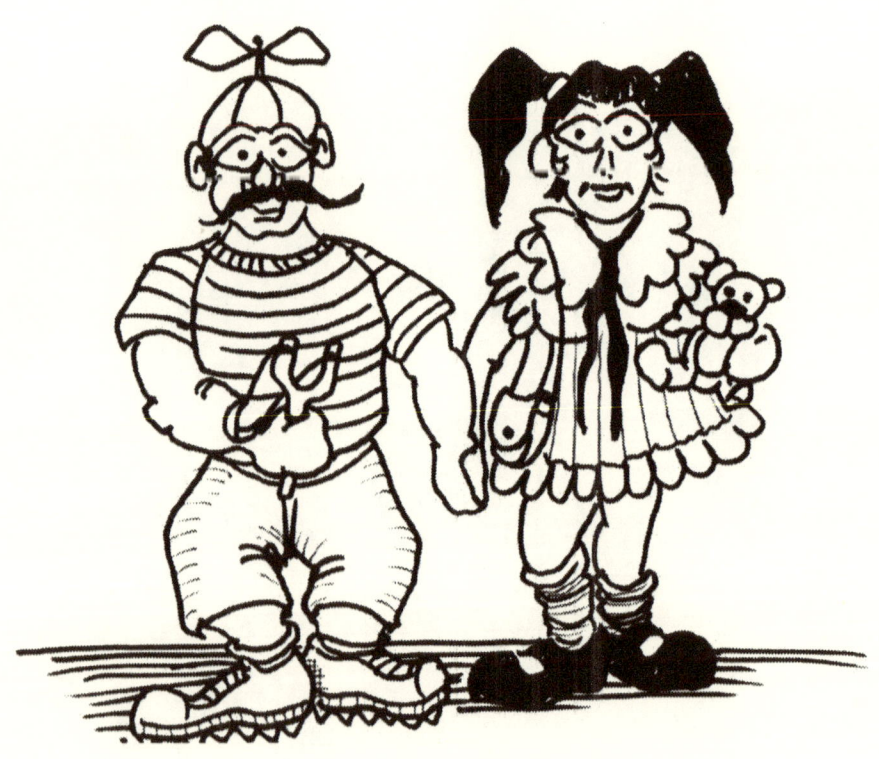

GROW UP

CHAPTER EIGHT

GROW UP

Who is responsible for your health, your life? When we are children our parents are responsible for us. As we grow up we need to learn to take more and more responsibility for ourselves until finally we become fully responsible. However, this process doesn't always happen for many of us. We learn responsibility in some aspects of our lives, but not in others. Life teaches us that we have to do certain things or else we face the consequences of not doing them. The law of cause and effect takes place. The laws of nature take over and we learn that what we do or do not do has some inevitable consequences. Some of us learn from these consequences and others repeat the same behavior and learn very little.

As a child, I, like many others, learned that when I was sick the doctor would get me well. So when we are young we are taught or conditioned to think that the doctor has the ability to cure us. I was not taught that my own body will help itself. I never realized that when I was sick it was my body that healed itself, not the doctor. I also learned that drugs would heal my illness and that antibiotics would kill the bacteria. My mind was trained to believe what my parents and society taught me about health. I never was taught anything about the cause of disease.

The sperm and the egg know what to do without the help of a doctor. The natural programming takes place according to the laws of nature which no doctor can reproduce.

As we become aware of more information, we are able to take more responsibility for our health. Getting more information and being more responsible go hand in hand. Does your medical doctor teach you how to eliminate the cause of your ill health, or just alleviate the symptom with drugs? How much influence do the pharmaceutical companies have on medical school education and on medical doctors? Where does the research money for new studies and drugs come from? How is the research conducted? These are just a few questions to examine. There are many more. Does a headache come from lack of aspirin? Why not find the causes of the headache so it doesn't recur?

When it comes down to the bottom line, there is no doctor that can be responsible for you. It doesn't matter if that doctor is an M.D., D.C., Ph. D., N.D., O.D., O.M., etc. No one can be responsible for you—only you, yourself. Taking on that responsibility is your job. If you don't choose to take it on, you are choosing the consequences. If you choose to educate yourself about your health you will benefit from the knowledge. Self-education is the foundation of good health. This is a lifelong process. A holistic team of doctors from various disciplines can be helpful in examining you from various points of view. However, such a team is not easy to find or work with, since the team members usually don't respect each other's discipline or communicate sufficiently with each other. Once again the responsibility comes back to you and the follow-through is yours. If you see various doctors you need to put all the pieces of information together and get feedback from the doctors.

If you lack information about your health or ill health, it is a function of the amount of responsibility you take for your self-education. Doctors don't know everything and can't be expected to. They are limited in their time and energy. Their first calling is to take care of themselves and of their lives, not of you. If your first priority is to take care of yourself, you will give it the time and effort your life deserves. What comes before your health? If your good health isn't your first priority, ask yourself what is, and then think about it! It's time to grow up!

What you can do

You need to take responsibility for your health and lifestyle. Remember that no one else can do it for you. Don't wait till you get sick to start taking responsibility. Overcome your conditioning about doctors and see them realistically, especially in time of need when you tend to put yourself in their hands. Do your own research and investigation of all options. Be responsible for educating yourself about the causes of disease and how to cleanse your body of toxins.   Live and work in a healthy environment.

Exercise

Read a book of your choice about health in the next two weeks and list ten things you have learned. Put five of them into practice in weeks three and four. How do you feel about yourself at the end of the month? Keep taking more responsibility for what ails you and search for the cause.

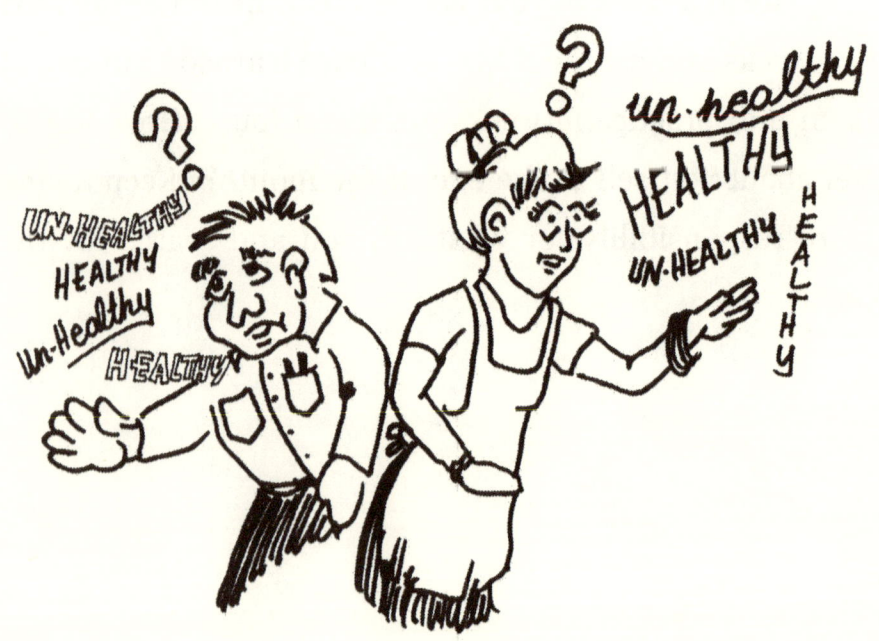

PRIORITIES

CHAPTER NINE

PRIORITIES

What is your first priority in life? Isn't it your life? Many people don't think about their life until it becomes threatened.   When this happens their focus changes. Someone with life-threatening cancer cannot stop thinking about it. Someone who has had a heart attack or a stroke can never forget about the devastating effects it has had on him/her. Illness changes your priorities and often the priorities of those around you.

When you look at the statistics of life-threatening diseases such as cancer and cardiovascular disease, how do you react? Do you think of yourself as a possible candidate for cancer, or do you ignore these statistics? When you know that cardiovascular disease is the number one cause of death in the United States, do you think it is a cause of personal concern or do you think it will not happen to you?

Why wait to become ill when so much knowledge is available about disease prevention? Do you have other priorities which seem to be more important at the moment? Each day, when you wake up in the morning, what is on your mind and what do you do? "Food, clothing and shelter" are basic for our daily survival. However, without good health we are limited in our pursuit of basic survival. Most of us in the United States have food, clothing and shelter. We then focus on acquiring and accumulating more and more. We spend most of our lives doing this, rather than spending enough time thinking about and practicing disease prevention. We know many Americans are overweight, but not sick enough to change their priorities.

In order to change priorities, you need to know what they are. If you make a list of your ten priorities in the order of importance, you would be able to evaluate them. Most people follow an automatic routine and are not aware of how they spend their time and energy. They go on day to day until the weekend and then change their behavior. When vacation time comes, they change their behavior again and then return to the day-to-day routine. How often do you stop to look at all of this? Where does your good health and disease prevention fit in? How often does it fit in during the week? What is your level of consciousness on a daily basis?

Once again nature's laws come into play and the cause and effect take place. Eat the wrong foods and you will have the effects over a period of time. So the choice of your priorities is yours. If you choose to look at yourself and your priorities you can evaluate and change them. If you choose to do nothing, you will keep getting what you have now. Think about it.

What you can do

Make good health your first priority and then act upon it. You know that without your good health everything else will stop. For those of you who are driven for more and more, ask yourself if your priorities need reviewing. Why wait to get sick before you change priorities?

Exercise

List ten priorities in your life in order of importance. The following day spend fifteen minutes reviewing their order and make any changes you want. Repeat this ten days later and then compare the list with the original one. Have you changed, have external circumstances changed, or have both changed?

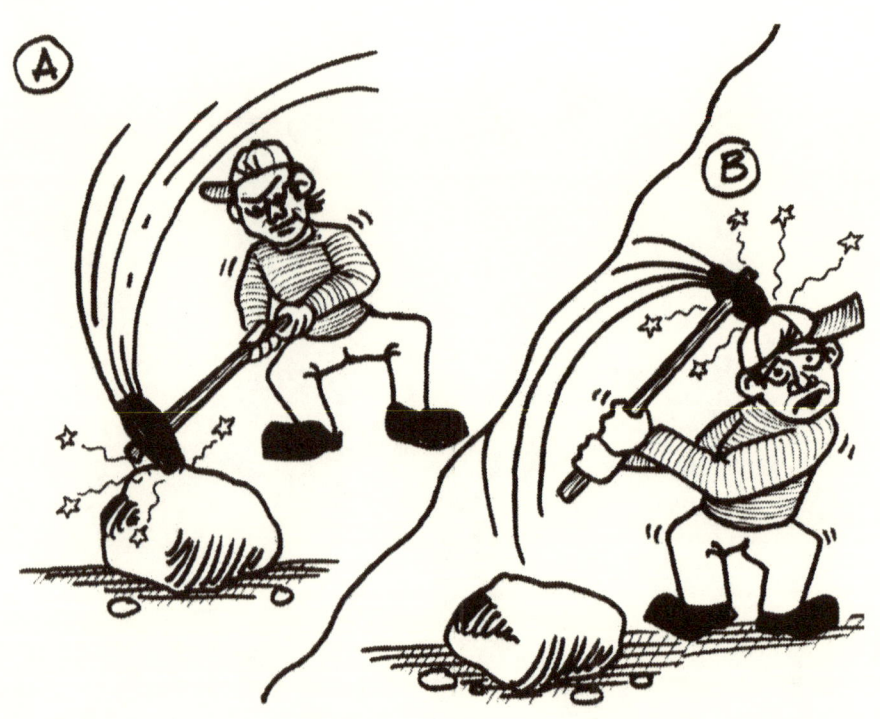

ARE YOU ANGRY?

CHAPTER TEN

ARE YOU ANGRY?

How often are you frustrated with something in your life? Frustration often leads to anger. Some people get angry easily and frequently. Sometimes anger can be unconscious anger. This takes place when something happens that angers you; however, you repress the feeling so that you don't feel it consciously. This mechanism of repression can also take place with other feelings.

When you are angry with yourself, you may also repress it so that it becomes unconscious. The energy of unconscious anger may often lead to self-destructive behavior. For example, people who bite their nails have developed an automatic habit. There are many kinds of self-destructive behavior. Many years ago I had a patient who was enraged at his father. His anger came out in his driving. He had eight auto accidents in nine months.

Self-destructive behavior may be one of the causes of being overweight. There are many ways in which people hurt themselves. They are aware of hurting themselves, yet go on doing it because they feel compelled by forces beyond their control. Each time, this mechanism of repressed anger turns into self-destructive behavior, and is repeated again and again, a pattern or habit develops. Each repetition strengthens the habit and it begins to feel as though this habit or behavior is out of your control. You just do it.

When you are the victim of your own self-destructive behavior it is very difficult to make changes because you are not aware of the whole mechanism. There are other mechanisms that also prevent change. In psychology we call these mechanisms defense mechanisms. Some that are commonly known are avoidance, procrastination, and denial. These three are rather simple to understand. When you avoid, procrastinate, or deny, you don't have to confront the issue. "Let's talk about it later," is one way of avoiding. "I don't know; I need more time to think it over," may be procrastination. "No, no, that's not true," may be a form of denial. There are many variations of these mechanisms which may prevent change.

These mechanisms have the impact of closing you down, so you are unable to change. If you examine yourself and find you have any of these processes going on in you, you may want to get professional help.

What you can do

How often do you get angry? Do you have any unhealthy habits that you would like to get rid of? Face yourself honestly and then examine why you are defending yourself or hurting yourself with self-destructive behavior.

Exercise

Count how many times you get angry in two weeks and observe your behavior when you are angry. Make a brief note about why you got angry and what you did. Did you do anything to hurt yourself or anyone else? Did you eat or drink anything after the anger episode? Was it healthy or unhealthy?

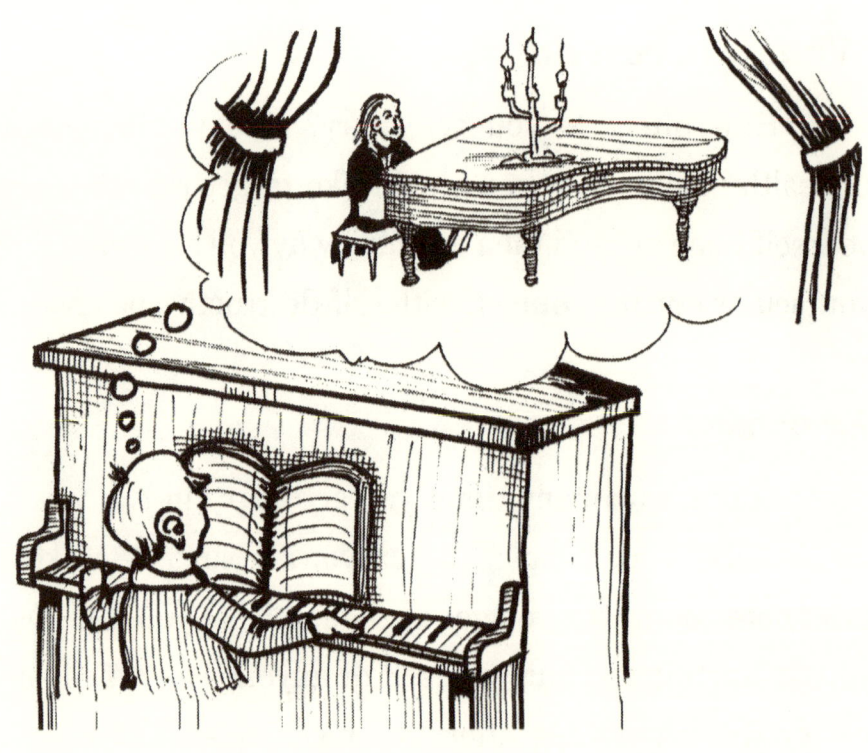

PRACTICE MAKES PERFECT

CHAPTER ELEVEN

"PRACTICE MAKES PERFECT"

The saying, "practice makes perfect" is well known. The more you practice the better you get is quite obvious. Practicing takes discipline and discipline is necessary to change your ways. Building discipline requires motivation and is a growth process. Learning discipline and patience go together. Discipline is learned from our parents, teachers, rules of society, etc. This kind of discipline is outwardly enforced. Self-discipline is something we enforce on ourselves because we are aware of the law of cause and effect.

If you have a goal you need to take the necessary steps to get there. If your goal is to get and use the knowledge available to live a healthier lifestyle, you need discipline. Some of us avoid self-discipline because it takes effort and it is easier to allow ourselves to escape making this effort. Each time you make the effort you gain; each time you avoid the effort you lose time in attaining your goal. The effort starts in your mind and thoughts. You are your own director; you program yourself and your life. You may have an inner struggle about doing something. I have one a few times in the evening after a busy day. I struggle with myself about making a large organic salad. I believe it is good for me to eat in rather than go out to eat food that is not as healthy. I stand in my kitchen deliberating about what do. Sometimes I am motionless for ten seconds, caught in my conflict: to go out or to stay in and make the salad. It's a battle. I give myself some logic by telling myself I have to drive to get to the restaurant and I know the food is not organically grown, and then I have to drive back. It will only take me about fifteen minutes to make the salad and I wouldn't be ingesting pesticides, fertilizers, hormones, etc. Yes, it is a struggle because I don't want to make the effort. However, each time I make the salad, it seems to get easier to do.

Somewhat opposite to discipline is self-indulgence or over-indulgence. I'm sure we all know what that means. Didn't you ever eat a whole pint of ice cream? You knew you should stop but you had a little bit more and a little bit more until you were close to the bottom, and then you thought that there was only a little bit left so you might as well finish it. Did a similar thing ever happen with champagne, wine, chocolate, or some food? Did you give yourself permission to overindulge yourself? This may be easier than stopping or may be very enjoyable at the moment. However, the law of cause and effect is inescapable and you will have the consequences.

Lack of discipline and over-indulgence both interfere with the ability to change.

What you can do

Discipline is a step-by-step growth process, starting with the easiest, smallest step that you can succeed with. Be consistent and persistent in your pursuit and make it part of your routine. You developed the discipline to brush your teeth every day. You can enhance your health when you make the decision to do it.

Exercise

Make fresh vegetable juice four days a week for two weeks. Chew your food until it liquefies in your mouth at dinner once a week for two weeks. Have you more discipline at the end of the second week or did you give up?

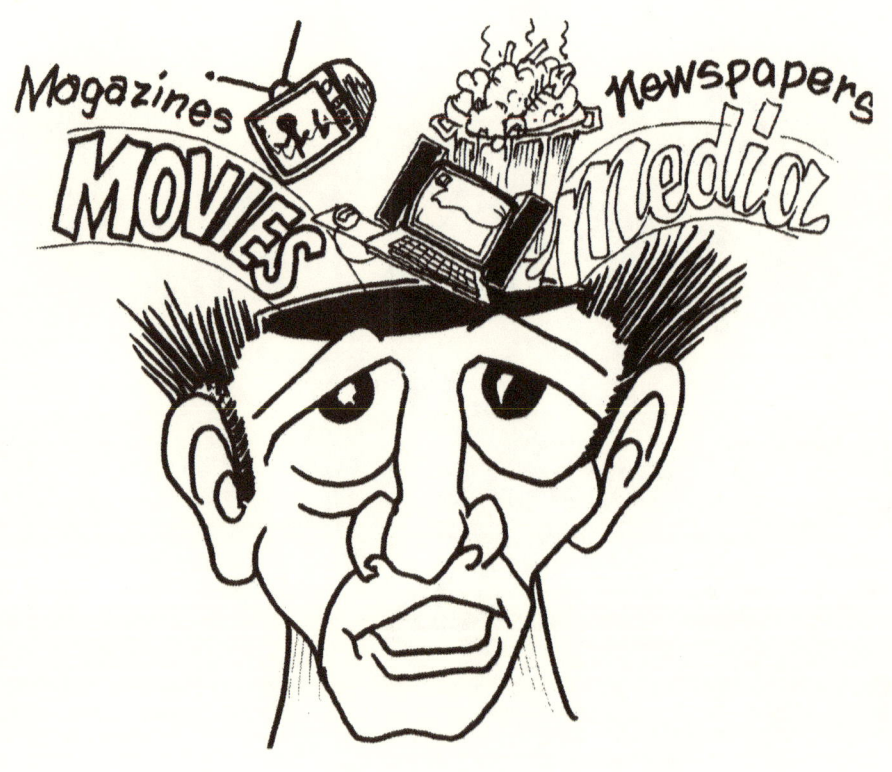

BRAINWASHED

CHAPTER TWELVE

BRAINWASHED

Psychological studies have shown that conditioning can take place prior to birth. From the day we are born we are being conditioned to many things in our environment and also taught to believe whatever our parents, teachers, relatives, religion, culture, etc., tell us. Some of these beliefs such as advertisements are not true. We are taught a certain amount of "false education" and illusions. As we repeat our beliefs they tend to become stronger, and many of us develop a defensive position when they are questioned.

Yes, we are "brainwashed." We now have over seven thousand medications that we believe "help" people become healthier. We tend to listen to the medical gods who prescribe them with very little questioning. We know there have been thousands of unnecessary surgeries. Some of us have almost become automatons and many of us lack self-reflection and awareness. Our daily routines have little or no thinking time about ourselves. We are caught up in our materialistic acquisitive world, which always has something new to offer. Some of us live for the weekend or for vacations. Some of us never have enough so we overwork to acquire more. Even those with millions and billions can't stop, and they are featured in magazines as idols. Some of us glorify movie stars and sports figures. Yes, we are "brainwashed."

With a mental set like this, following the herd, how can we think about changing to a healthier lifestyle? It is very difficult. When some of us attempt to change we feel uncomfortable about giving up what we like to do. Others feel anxiety because certain habits (food, drinks) we have comfort us. Eating often has an emotional component as well as a physical one. I can remember when I was a sixth grade teacher and had to drive to work from New York City to Orangeburg. It was only seventeen miles away. I always carried chocolate bars in my car for security and ate some on the way to work. I was no different from anyone else who was eating for emotional reasons. At that time I had no awareness of why I needed the chocolate and the Hagen Daz ice cream I ate at home. I couldn't even think about changing since I didn't perceive any problem. My "tranquilizers" were just part of my normal routine. My underlying anxiety about my loneliness was totally buried at that time.

Some beliefs have become so strong that they are put into law. In the state of California the only legal treatments for cancer are radiation, chemotherapy and surgery. Any other treatments are a felony, and the doctor is fined $10,000, goes to jail, and loses his/her license! How far can "brainwashing" go? When we are brainwashed, it is difficult to change.

What you can do

Examine and evaluate things that you are told by others or that are advertised in the media. Make sure that you are satisfied with your personal investigations before you take action. Think things out for yourself after you hear the "pitch."

Exercise

Choose one advertisement for food or a drug that you have heard on TV and spend one hour a week investigating its effects for the next two weeks. If you have used any drug in the last three years, study it and find out its side effects and if it eliminates the cause of the problem or relieves the symptoms of a deeper problem.

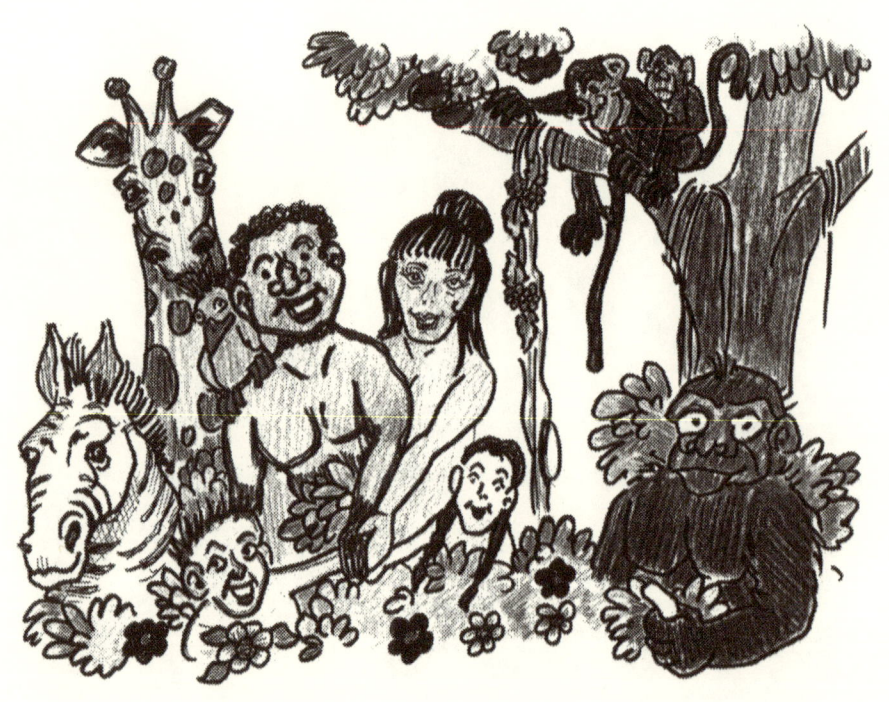

WHAT CAN YOU DO?

CHAPTER THIRTEEN

WHAT CAN YOU DO?

Do you want to live long or die young? Do you want your children to get more childhood cancer, diabetes, etc., and die young? Do you want to slowly kill planet Earth? It's all up to YOU and only you—not our government, politicians, the FDA, the EPA, the multi-national corporations or the powers that be, or even your medical doctor and the drug companies. You pay money for products that will help you and your children die prematurely. Only you can change yourself. If you continue to believe that you are taken care of by the government, multinational corporations, drug companies, and your doctor, you will not only continue to get what you have now, but will get sicker even faster than ever. More money is spent on cloning than on educating our children about the causes of disease.

If you continue to believe that you are helpless you will remain helpless. It's up to you, one by one, to make the changes in your lifestyle that will give you the power to influence and destroy those who are slowly destroying you.

You can wake up or stay asleep until it hits you in the face, and when it does you can go for your bypass, surgery, radiation, chemotherapy, or drugs. You can reduce the risk of a heart attack or even eliminate it by proper diet and lifestyle, or try Merck's last drug, Zocor, and suffer the side effects. Plavix, a drug being advertised on TV, is to prevent a second heart attack. Wouldn't it be better to find the cause of the first one and change your lifestyle?

What would be helpful is a clear, calm mind that is willing to take responsibility for yourself, your children, and the Earth. We are all connected to nature and are not separate from it or "above it." When we understand that we are a part of nature and use this awareness to our benefit by living in harmony with it, we will stop destroying the trees, the animals, the birds, the fish, the oxygen in the air, the soil, and each other.

The self-interests of certain individuals and groups who never have enough money or power are destroying you, nature, and the human spirit. This destruction must be stopped. We need to wake up and protect our children and ourselves, for we are responsible for the future. When we begin to change our individual lifestyle, we begin to change our environment. Materialism is not a substitute for love. We cannot fill our hearts with things; we cannot raise our spirits without love.

Did you know cancer costs were about $103 billion a year in 1990, according to the National Cancer Institute?

Did you know that the Harvard Department of Nutrition has received funding from McDonald's Corp., Armour & Co., Coca-Cola Co., Kellogg Co., Sugar Association, Hershey Foods, Oscar Meyer Co., etc., according to "Adventures in Nutrition Appendix 6"? Other sources of funding are Abbott Laboratories, Eli Lilly and Co., Merck, Sharp and Dohme, Parke-Davis and Co., Pfizer, Inc., etc., as well as from the Council for Tobacco Research and the Tobacco Industries Research Foundation.

Did you know that in 1989 restaurant TV advertising was $1.2 billion, with McDonald's spending $425 million and Burger King, KFC, Pizza Hut, Taco Bell, Wendy's, etc., spending the rest? Did you know that according to the

1992 World Almanac and Book of Facts, the alcohol, food and tobacco advertising is about $5.7 billion a year?

When we oppose the laws of nature we create illness. What we eat and drink affects the quality of our blood and nervous system, e.g. the over-consumption of salt causes constriction in tissues, nerves, and vessels. We must always understand the cause of the disease and never be satisfied with just treating the symptoms.

The importance of a proper lifestyle cannot be overemphasized. Lifestyle is a total of all our thoughts, emotions, behavior, diet, etc., on a 24/7 basis. Lifestyle is the major contributor to disease. It is the total of all our functioning. Our body functions as a totality, not in separate pieces. Our body has a natural healing power if given what it needs to do so. It does not need processed or preserved food, food that is depleted in enzymes, or food grown on depleted soil.

Now is the time for you to start eating organically grown fruits and vegetables. They are more nutritious, taste much better, and will help keep you healthy. Organic food is grown without the use of synthetic fertilizers, pesticides, fungicides or herbicides, and is processed without irradiation.

Let's change "Managed Care" to "Managed Prevention" and become more concerned with our "Gross National Health" that our "Gross National Product." Wake up, America!

What you can do

You can make a decision to choose a healthy lifestyle. You can stop feeding yourself and your children toxic food. You can have an effect on the environment when you change your lifestyle. You can ask your doctor to find the cause of your disease and not treat the symptom. Yon can have the courage to overcome all obstacles in the way to good health. You can value your good health as the most important thing in your life. Educate yourself!

THINK ABOUT IT

If you think about it

You'll begin to tout it

Society gets worse

It's mankind's new curse

Destroying ourselves

No more little elves

As pollution increases

Natural living ceases

The air goes bad

Oh it's so sad

The soil is depleted

We are all very cheated

Pesticides and sprays

Will shorten our days

Creating more drugs

Killing all the bugs

But new ones grow

They win the show

Rivers are unclean

Garbage dumps are seen

More money for the rich
Isn't it time to switch
From those who control
We all pay the toll
With more disease
Losing the trees
Paying trillions
Killing millions
Pretending not to know
The right way we must go
Stop the greed
Plant the seed
We must live together
Like birds of a feather
If not our children will die
We all know the reason why
Unless we stop now
And to nature bow
The earth will begin to end
The corporations must bend
We must change our ways

DO YOU HAVE THE COURAGE TO CHANGE?

And create good days
If you think about it
You'll begin to tout it.

WHERE ARE YOU GOING?

Where are you going

Without you knowing?

You travel so fast

Will you ever last?

From point A to B

Nothing do you see

From point C to D

Little left of thee

Then faster you go

Surely you don't know

As you travel on your way

Doing the same thing each day

If you could stop a bit

And in your good chair sit

And become aware

If only you dare

To think some more

And find the door

Where are you going

Without you knowing?

BIBLIOGRAPHY

Allen, J., "As a Man Thinketh," Barnes and Noble, 1992, ISBN 0-8802-9785-0

Ausubel, K., "When Healing Becomes a Crime," Healing Arts Press, 2000, ISBN 0-89281-925-1

Bogdanovich, R., M.D., "The Cause is the Cure," Spirit Spring Foundation, 2001, ISBN 0-9704403-0-9

Epstein, S., "The Politics of Cancer Revisited," East Ridge Press, 1998, ISBN 0-914896-46-6

Gerson, M., M.D. "A Cancer Therapy," Whittier Books, 1958, ISBN 0-88268-203-2

Harris, W., M.D., "The Scientific Basis of Vegetarianism," Hawaii Health Publishers, 1415 Victoria St., Suite 1106, Honolulu, HI 96822-3663, 1995, ISBN 0-9646538-0-X

Lopez, D.A., M.D., Williams, R.M., M.D., Ph.D., Miehlke, K., M.D., "Enzymes, the Fountain of Life," The Neville Press, 1994, ISBN 1-884303-00-5

Rapp, D.J., M.D., "Is This Your Child's World?" Bantam Books, 1996, ISBN 0-553-10513-2

Robbins, J., "The Food Revolution," Conari Press, 2001, ISBN 1-57324-702-2

Urban, Walter J., "Integrative Therapy: Foundations of Holistic and Self Healing" Guild of Tutors Press, 1978, ISBN 89615-00406

ABOUT THE AUTHOR

Walter J. Urban, Ph. D., is a research psychoanalyst registered with the Medical Board of California. His registration number is RP7 (the seventh one in the state). He was the director of the Theodore Reik Consultation Center in New York and on the Board of Directors of the National Psychological Association for Psychoanalysis, the American Psychotherapy Association, and the Gerson Institute. He was a consultant on a National Institute of Mental Health grant and author of the column entitled "Lifestyle Psychotherapy" in the Annals of the American Psychotherapy Association, where he was a Fellow. He is a member of the American Psychological Association and the California State Psychological Association and many other professional organizations.

Dr. Walter J. Urban is the originator of Integrative Therapy. His book "Integrative Therapy: Foundation for Holistic and Self Healing" was published in 1978.

Dr. Urban was host and producer of the first psychological television talk show in 1976 entitled "Psychoanalysis."

Now he is first again with this unique approach to better health and disease prevention. There are many books filled with good information about health. Most people find it difficult to use this information in their lives on a daily basis because making the necessary changes is very difficult.

This book reveals the twelve basic reasons why people don't change. Understanding these obstacles is the first step to overcoming them. These obstacles are explained in simple, everyday language, and each chapter has an exercise to help you overcome the obstacle.

It is a must read for everyone who wants to live a longer, healthier life. It's another first in its field!

This book is a breakthrough book and the first of its kind. It focuses on specific reasons why people don't change. Understanding the obstacles through a conscious awareness makes it easier for people to take the responsibility to change. Many people offer reasons or "excuses" for maintaining the status quo. They seldom look in the mirror and confront their issues and then challenge themselves to make the changes that they know would create a healthier lifestyle. If you don't change for the better, you will keep heading in the same direction and probably get worse. Your old habits and patterns are reinforced each day and become harder and harder to change. That's why the book offers simple suggestions of what you can do to start the changing process today. These exercises will get you on the right track and help you develop discipline and new habits in which you take more responsibility for your greater well being.

There are no other books like this one. Other books tell you what you should do to live a healthier lifestyle, but lack the self confronting issues that are clearly and simply presented in this book. With this in mind the benefits of "Do You Have The Courage To Change" cannot be found anywhere else.

www.ingramcontent.com/pod-product-compliance
Lightning Source LLC
Chambersburg PA
CBHW030341290526
45785CB00004B/1554